Table of Contents

Preface	2
Introduction	4
Chapter 1: The Comprehensive Care Team	13
Chapter 2: Pharmacological Treatment	33
Chapter 3: Physical Therapy	49
Chapter 4: Alternative and Adjunctive Methods	73
Chapter 5: Fall Prevention Programs	118
Chapter 6: PD Staples and Conclusion	133
Resource Guide Consolidated Index	139
References	143

Field Guide for Parkinson's

Preface

Field Guide for Parkinson's

There will be a variety of resources in this book including a list of sources accessed and websites but also through QR codes to allow for quick and easy access while reading. If you're unfamiliar with how to use a QR code, simply open the camera of your phone and adjust so that the code is within the camera. A link will pop up that you can select, which will then take you to the location.

https://support.apple.com/en-us/HT208843

Field Guide for Parkinson's

Introduction

Field Guide for Parkinson's

Parkinson's disease is a very common neurological condition and is second in prevalence only to Alzheimer's disease, affecting 2% of individuals over the age of 65. Because of its widespread impact, you surely have some prior knowledge or recognition of the condition but regardless, the following information is provided as a quick summary.[1]

Parkinson's disease (PD) is a chronic condition of the brain characterized by four primary symptoms, described as "clinical syndrome features". These symptoms are rigidity, bradykinesia (slowness of movement), resting tremors, and postural instability. Besides these symptoms, there are other common signs including both motor (related to movement) and non-motor, including things such as micrographia (small, cramped handwriting), anxiety/depression, taste/smell changes, trouble sleeping, and difficulty with speech and swallowing. Initial symptoms that may include loss of smell, constipation, orthostatic hypotension (significant decrease in blood pressure when transitioning to

Field Guide for Parkinson's

standing from either a sitting position or lying down), changes in mood, or sleep disturbances, namely a disruption in REM sleep.[1] The Parkinson's disease that we refer to in this book, and the condition named after its discoverer, James Parkinson, who in 1817 described the condition first as "the shaking palsy", discusses cases of unknown etiology (idiopathic).[1] While the exact cause of common idiopathic Parkinson's is unknown (hence the descriptor "idiopathic"), it is thought that environment and genetics play a role. For those with early-onset Parkinson's disease, occurring before the age of 40, the cause may be related to genetics more so than late-onset which occurs after the age of 40. Some known factors that are related to diagnosis of Parkinson's disease include viruses (encephalitis lethargica), toxins (carbon monoxide), certain medications, tumors, and other conditions. Furthermore, Parkinsonian-like symptoms can present from other degenerative conditions of the brain.[1,2]

Field Guide for Parkinson's

Within the brain there is a group of nuclei known as the basal ganglia. One component of the basal ganglia, the substantia nigra, contains neurons responsible for releasing dopamine, a messenger molecule that plays an important role in movement, mood, and pleasure. Too little dopamine results in muscular stiffness, tremors, difficulty eating and swallowing whereas too much dopamine, which could occur in a contrasting condition of the basal ganglia such as Huntington's Disease, results in jerky or writhing movements (followed by rigidity in later stages).[1,2,3,4]

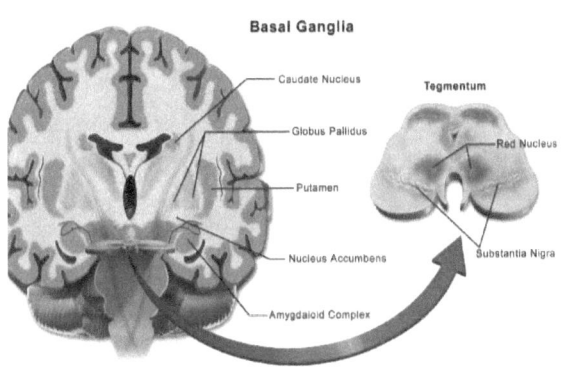

https://www.wikiwand.com/en/Basal_ganglia

Field Guide for Parkinson's

Rigidity may exist unilaterally at first but eventually spread to both sides. Concentration on a movement during its occurrence may lead to a higher degree of rigidity. This presents through the difficulty initiating and terminating movements. Between the time of initiation and termination of the movement, the spinal cord and cerebellum take over, mediating our unconscious movements as observable through the capability to keep moving rhythmically after the initial hurdle of beginning the movement. As we'll discuss later, this is why therapeutic techniques that manipulate where our attention is during movement through modalities such as music are popular.

Bradykinesia (or slowness of movement) is another one of the cardinal features of Parkinson's disease as mentioned previously. Rather than resulting solely from weakness or because of tremors, the bradykinesia exhibited with PD happens because of the insufficient recruitment of musculature as signaled through the brain (in the basal ganglia). Because the mind is unable to internally generate movements effectively, resulting in their small magnitude or slow execution, external cueing can be of assistance through things such as vision or sound, as evident in many of the exercises suggested for those with PD.[1]

Tremors, the third main feature of Parkinson's exist only at rest initially, with a majority happening in the hands in a "pill rolling" rolling fashion. They may be worsened when in a more anxious, stressed, or excited state. In the later stages of Parkinson's disease the tremors may continue with movements.[1]

The final of the four primary motor presentations of Parkinson's is postural instability. A decreased ability to maintain the center of mass of one's body within the base of support exists in those with PD. This is apparent especially when balance is perturbed, through difficulty re-stabilizing because of the improper recruitment of muscle fibers as previously mentioned. Postural righting reactions that happen at the hips and ankles or through taking steps are impaired because of this abnormal coactivation of musculature, where the body tends to lock-up rather than adjust and regain balance.[1]

These features typically manifest at least 5 years after the onset of PD, but are the most widely recognized symptoms and therefore can result in a delayed diagnosis. The first symptom in between 13-33% of patients is gait disturbances and/or postural instability. This is commonly displayed through stooped posture, difficulty with changes in direction, and festination of gait; where the step frequency progressively increases while the stride length decreases cite the book. Difficulty swallowing, soft speech with poor articulation, slowed thinking, and constipation are other symptoms that are exhibited in those with PD and should be looked for more frequently to avoid delayed diagnosis. Because of this, researchers with the Movement Disorder Society sought to provide better diagnostic criteria to help clinical diagnosis which include a larger set of symptoms to

Field Guide for Parkinson's

observe, criteria to rule out PD, and different levels of certainty based on the presenting symptoms.[1,5]

Next, we'll look into the medical professionals and other professions that are there to work together with you. We'll discuss the common medical management strategies, classification, and then transition to a focused view of the role of physical therapy. The following is a detailed overview of Parkinson's disease that can be accessed through the QR code provided on the next page.

Field Guide for Parkinson's

<u>RESOURCE ITEM #1:</u> *PD Explained*

https://www.khanacademy.org/science/health-and-medicine/nervous-system-diseases/parkinsons-disease/

Field Guide for Parkinson's

Chapter 1

The Comprehensive Care Team

Field Guide for Parkinson's

An interdisciplinary approach is important to implement because of the long-term and variety of systems and functions that PD affects. One study by Dr. Christopher Goetz, published in the journal of movement disorders and referred to in the everyday health newsletter, reports that treatment outcomes for those with Parkinson's disease may be better when a neurologist, nurse, movement disorder specialist, and social worker are involved in treatment.[6] Who is this movement disorder specialist that he mentions? According to the APTA, "physical therapists are movement experts who improve quality of life through prescribed exercise, hands-on care, and patient education."[7]

Today, to practice as a physical therapist in the United States, you must earn a doctor of physical therapy degree from an accredited institution, where as a student physical therapist the individual becomes proficient in their understanding of biology/anatomy, exercise physiology, pathophysiology, biomechanics, kinesiology, neuroscience, pharmacology, behavioral sciences, reasoning, evidence-based practice, musculoskeletal practice, cardiovascular and pulmonary, endocrine, metabolic, and sociology/ethics/values. Not only do physical therapists assist through the process of recovering from injuries to things like joints, ligaments, etc., but they are well-versed in conditions affecting other bodily systems such as conditions affecting the brain; i.e. PD. Before discussing this deeper, let's turn our attention to some of the other members that are included in a multidisciplinary treatment team.

Neurologist

Neurologists are specialist physicians who are the go-to contact for coordinating and assisting with major decision making throughout the course of Parkinson's. Some may even further specialize within the scope of neurology, focusing specifically on conditions such as PD or other movement disorders. Referrals to other medical professionals regarding prescription medications and therapy in the form of physical therapy, occupational, therapy, or speech therapy (although direct access without a referral may be possible in some cases) are done with the guidance of a trusted Neurologist. The following QR code and link lead to a database of neurologists throughout the country which could be beneficial in the search of one, if not already considered.[6]

Field Guide for Parkinson's

RESOURCE ITEM #2: *Neurologist Database*

https://www.healthgrades.com/neurology-directory

As previously stated, neurologists can further specialize within their field, focusing on movement pathologies and earning titles such as a movement disorder specialist (MDS). MDS have extensive knowledge of the therapies and ongoing research of PD and can be found through the directory accessible through RESOURCE ITEM #3 seen on the following page. The physicians included in this list are active members of the International Parkinson and Movement Disorder Society, but this resource is not an exhaustive list of all members within this society since MDS membership is voluntary and not required to be a specialist of movement disorders.[8,9]

Field Guide for Parkinson's

RESOURCE ITEM #3: *MDS Database*

https://mds.movementdisorders.org/directory/

Field Guide for Parkinson's

Physician's Assistant

Primary care physicians also play a role in the coordination of care, specifically focusing on your overall health and well-being in terms of the non-movement-related symptoms that PD can produce and other traditional reasons for doctor visits such as vaccinations, illnesses, etc. Similarly, a physician assistant may serve this role for you in some clinics and can potentially be more accessible because of the shortage of physicians, especially in rural settings.[10]

Nurses

Nurses have a critical role in the healthcare field and have a wide variety and reach within it. From the hospital to the home, they are a valuable resource for individuals with any number of different conditions and assist with anything ranging from administering medications to supporting transitions of care. A specialization in Parkinson's for nurses has existed since 1989 and has been progressively growing since.[11] These nurses have invaluable advice and support to those with PD in addition to the already important role that they provide through their traditional nursing field of knowledge. In addition to the traditional Parkinson's specialization, the Parkinson's Foundation recently began a 1-year fellowship program for training and supporting nurses who desire to specialize in PD, where they will receive mentorship, research experience, and training in order to build a community of Parkinson's nurse experts to provide the best patient-specific care possible.[12]

<u>*Occupational Therapists*</u>

Occupational therapists (OT) also serve a significant role, with a focus on fine motor activities such as cooking, hygiene, dressing, and other skills that require precision and accurate movements. These individuals can have a massive impact because of their ability to provide therapeutic interventions focused on things that you might find integral to your personal life through hobbies like playing cards, quilting, gardening or independence with things like tying shoes or putting on a belt. Short-term intensive sessions with an OT which focus on specific individual goals are supported by current research on the matter, although the body of evidence on OT for PD alone, not in conjunction with other therapies, is sparse.[13]

Speech Therapists

Speech-language pathologists are an essential part to the care management team to address impairments with speech volume/articulation and swallowing.[6] One Parkinson's specific specialization that exists within this profession is the LSVT (Lee Silverman Voice Treatment) Loud Certification. Through the LSVT LOUD and LSVT BIG exercises, which will be mentioned in the upcoming physical therapy section, improvements in speech and movement speed and amplitude can be seen in both the short and long-term.[14,15] Speech therapy should be initiated even before noticing changes in communication to delay and mitigate changes in voice and speech. In addition to focuses on speech and movement via speech and physical therapists, occupational therapists may also obtain LSVT certification. Coursework in the LSVT program includes fundamental treatment principles, treatment elements and exercise, customized treatment delivery for different stages of PD, techniques for assessment, and data and research supporting the treatments.[16] The resource on the next page gives an overview and examples of some of the LSVT LOUD and LSVT BIG treatment principles and execution.

Field Guide for Parkinson's

***RESOURCE ITEM #4:** LSVT Explained*

https://davisphinneyfoundation.org/lsvt-big-loud/

Dietician

Dieticians can be of assistance with food preparation and suggestions to allow for a sustainable dietary plan throughout the course of PD. With certain common Parkinson's medications such as L-dopa, diets high in protein can be detrimental to the drug's effectiveness because the amino acids that form proteins compete with L-dopa absorption during digestion. To counteract this issue, diets higher in calories and low in protein are typically advised with a general protein percentage of no more than 15%. Adjusting the time of day where protein is consumed the most to a time that is expected to be less physically active is another way to adjust for this drug-food interaction.[6] If you would like aide in the tedious task of formulating a diet that adheres to these suggested amounts, consult a registered dietician. The following link is a search tool to find a registered dietitian nutritionist near you.

Field Guide for Parkinson's

RESOURCE ITEM #5: *Dietician Search*

https://www.eatright.org/find-an-expert

Field Guide for Parkinson's

Mental Health Professionals

Psychologists, Therapists, and Neuropsychologists are members of the treatment team that can be overlooked as their effects are not seen through management of physical signs and symptoms or functional management of the condition but rather through mental and emotional well-being. Psychologist's role in health care has grown and, consequently, so has their understanding of disease-specific psychological effects and ability to practice in a manner that adopts this biopsychosocial approach, integrating both mental and physical health into interrelated aspects.[17] Through training, psychologists can obtain specialist certifications to become neuropsychologists through postdoctoral training as outlined via the American Board of Clinical Neuropsychology.[18] These professionals have an even deeper knowledge and understanding neurological conditions and address the relationship between the mind and the symptoms of PD.[6]. To find a board-certified clinical neuropsychologist, refer to the following link to a directory provided by the American Academy of Clinical Neuropsychology.

Field Guide for Parkinson's

RESOURCE ITEM #6: *Neuropsychologist directory*

https://theaacn.org/directory/

Field Guide for Parkinson's

Social Worker

Already, there have been numerous health professionals that have been mentioned as integral or possible members of a treatment team. With all of these members, and those that have yet to be mentioned, organizing who, how, when, and where to utilize these individuals can be dizzying (and expensive). A social worker is one way to address the logistical questions that may not be able to be answered by just one of these professionals and can be a resource-of-resources per-se, helping to navigate and sift through things like insurance, prescription plans, home devices and equipment.[6]

Pharmacist

One of the major first-line medical management treatments of Parkinson's disease is pharmacological treatment. There are a variety of different medications that work at various locations within the brain and body with functions designed to counteract both the central effects that Parkinson's disease has at the level of the brain, as well as to address the symptoms of the condition as they present. Medications for treating PD will be prescribed by either a neurologist or other MD but pharmacists are able to explain the purpose of the medications, instruct on how to take them/assist in organization when multiple medications are prescribed, and determine whether there are any interactions between the drugs or side effects that warrant attention.[6]

This chapter we have looked at a charcuterie of different health care workers and specialists that are trained to be of assistance to you throughout life in minimizing the effects and concerns of PD. With physicians, physician's assistants, nurses, occupational and speech therapists, nutritionists, psychologists, social workers and pharmacists, there are numerous people available to help and provide a multi-faceted approach towards the management of Parkinson's. With all of those professions having been mentioned, one important field of professionals, physical therapy, has yet to be discussed in depth. Before diving into physical therapy for

Parkinson's and its role and importance, we will look, next, at the pharmacological management that we began to inspect at the end of this chapter.

Field Guide for Parkinson's

Chapter 2

Pharmacological Treatment

Field Guide for Parkinson's

To prevent the rate of progression of Parkinson's, pharmacological management is essential. Whereas this perspective is not written by a pharmacist but rather through the lens of physical therapy, the knowledge of pharmacology is imperative across the interdisciplinary care-team and not limited only to those providing the prescriptions. The medication list can quickly become complex and challenging to sustain but is important for preventing large peaks and valleys in terms of severity of symptoms. Taking the medications at the same time every day, on a fixed schedule is one way to prevent missing doses and introducing the undesirable results that might occur. This can also prevent any difficulty that might be increased by waiting too long between doses and allowing for the effects of the previous medication to wear off. Another way to reduce the likelihood of forgetting a dose is through filling out a medication form to keep in your free Aware in Care kit which is available through the National Parkinson Foundation and can be found through the code presenting on the following page followed by the full kit. Having this information in one form can help ensure that the different health professionals on the same page.[1]

Field Guide for Parkinson's

RESOURCE ITEM #7: *Medication Form*

https://www.parkinson.org/sites/default/files/AIC-MedicationsForm2019.pdf

Field Guide for Parkinson's

RESOURCE ITEM #8: *Aware in Care kit*

https://www.parkinson.org/Living-with-Parkinsons/Resources-and-Support/Patient-Safety-Kit/Kit-Contents

Field Guide for Parkinson's

The no. 1, go-to, gold standard drug therapy used for Parkinson's disease was produced initially in the early 1961 before becoming widely used clinically by the end of the decade. This medication is Levodopa or L-dopa, and is commonly combined with carbidopa which provides assistance by allowing more levodopa to be absorbed in the brain.[1] L-dopa is a chemical precursor to dopamine, which is deficient in PD, and thus L-dopa seeks to offset this shortage through providing more of this pre-dopamine substance which is metabolized into dopamine within the brain. By this mechanism, levodopa is classified as a dopamine replacement medication. Carbidopa is essential for the effectiveness of L-dopa because of the high rate of metabolization of l-dopa before it is able to reach the target site in the brain. The drug Sinament represents the most common form of this levodopa/carbidopa combination and is available in an immediate-release and controlled-release forms to allow for the ability to control how often they must be administered, with the immediate-release form requiring multiple doses per day. Two of the four primary motor symptoms associated with Parkinson's are targeted with levodopa, with those symptoms being rigidity and bradykinesia. Upon the initiation of levodopa, reductions in these symptoms may be seen almost immediately during the "honeymoon period". The effectiveness of this medication typically lasts between 4-6 years which means that while it is a fantastic medication to implement, it cannot be the only answer because of this small window of success. There are also multiple adverse effects that may occur, especially during the latter stages of levodopa usage such as dyskinesia (involuntary or uncontrolled movements) or dystonias (involuntary contractions of muscles for a prolonged period). To counteract this, other medications may be administered during the wearing off period.[1]

While levodopa helps address symptoms of Parkinson's by adding more dopamine (through providing a precursor of it), dopamine agonists are another class of drug that seeks to improve the utilization of dopamine at the site which it is received. This class of medications may be initiated early in the disease process as a first line of defense and can be combined with levodopa to increase both dopamine availability and the reception of it. One benefit of dopamine agonists such as the drugs Pergolide and Bromocriptine, is that there is not a 4-6 year of effectiveness window as seen with levodopa, but instead, these drugs can be utilized long-term, alone, or in conjunction with other medications like levodopa. Side effects of dopamine agonists are most commonly nausea, sedation, constipation, dizziness, and hallucinations.[1]

The final main group of medications that focus on the brain's response to dopamine is monoamine oxidase inhibitors. Monoamine oxidase type B (MAO-B) is an enzyme that breaks down dopamine in the brain.[11] With early implementation of a monoamine oxidase B inhibitors, namely Selegiline, disease progression may be slowed.[1,19] They may be used alone, early after diagnoses or in conjunction with other PD medications. When used with l-dopa, smaller doses may be used. In addition to

Field Guide for Parkinson's

Selegiline (a.k.a. Deprenyl), another common MAO-B inhibitor is rasagiline (Azilect).[1] Possible adverse effects of monoamine oxidase type B inhibitors are dry mouth, nausea, orthostatic hypotension, confusion, hallucinations, and insomnia.[19]

In summary, dopamine utilization is addressed primarily through these three medication classes. Levodopa serves as the precursor to dopamine, therefore acting by providing more dopamine in the brain. Dopamine agonists help by increasing the sensitivity of dopamine receptor sites. Finally, MAO-B inhibitors aid in increasing dopamine's effects through preventing its breakdown. By providing more dopamine, increasing the sensitivity of the receptors of dopamine, and preventing dopamine from being broken down, these medications take an effective, multidimensional approach.[1]

Aside from working within the central nervous system, targeting dopamine production or utilization, another class of drugs focuses peripherally on symptom reduction. Nerve conduction to initiate movement at the site of a muscle requires a neurotransmitter called acetylcholine. A class of drugs known as anticholinergics counteract this signaling preventing motion and are useful for treatment of the tremors that occur with Parkinson's.[1] They also can assist in reducing dystonia and therefore might be used in conjunction with drugs that have dystonia as a side effect like the aforementioned, levodopa. Side effects of this class of medications are dry mouth, nausea/vomiting, blurred vision, confusion, and dizziness.

These are the most commonly applied medicinal treatments of Parkinson's disease. Because of its global impact on individuals, PD is a large topic of research and clinical trials are constantly being performed to find novel medicinal treatments. But as we've already discussed when talking about the numerous health professionals involved in a PD treatment team, a multifaceted approach is needed which also applies in the realm of the modalities that are applied. Pharmacological treatment cannot be the only form of treatment, at least with today's available medications. Another effective treatment of PD exists in the form of deep brain stimulation (DBS). This is a particularly effective treatment for those with advanced Parkinson's and works through blocking nerve signals in the basal ganglia within the brain that result in symptoms. In this modality, electrodes are implanted in the brain which have been calibrated to deliver a particular amount of current as controlled through a remote. In total, there are four parts that make up the deep brain stimulation system: the remote, electrodes implanted in the basal ganglia, a small device called a pulse generator that causes the electrical pulses similar to a pacemaker, and connecting leads between the electrodes and the device on the surface.[11] When pharmacological treatments of tremors becomes ineffective, improvements through the utilization of deep brain stimulation in nearly every patient with many experiencing almost total reduction in tremors and dyskinesias.[1] The symptoms of PD such as akinesia, rigidity, impaired gait speed and weakness may also be reduced although the responses are less prominent that the significant reductions in dyskinetic movements and tremors. Normal surgical risks apply to the procedure involving the implantation of these electrodes and other potential side effects including confusion, headache, falling/gait abnormalities, and speech disturbances exist but nonetheless, deep brain stimulation remains a reliable medical intervention for those with advanced Parkinson's or who are resistant to the aforementioned medicinal treatments.[20] Similar to this concept is transcranial direct current stimulation (tDCS) which has evidence backing its utilization for decreasing dyskinesias.[21] On the following page, an image representation can be seen of the deep brain stimulation system. Following this image, a QR code link to a video explanation of deep brain stimulation can be accessed.

Field Guide for Parkinson's

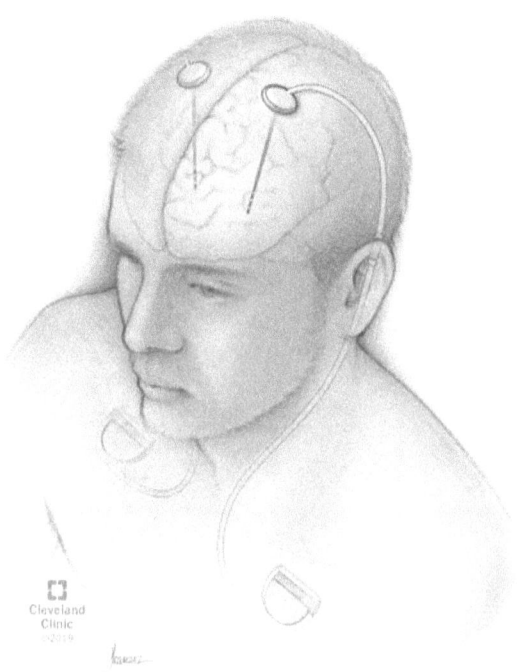

Deep Brain Stimulation.

https://my.clevelandclinic.org/health/treatments/4080-deep-brain-stimulation-for-parkinsons-disease-patients

Field Guide for Parkinson's

RESOURCE ITEM #9: Deep Brain Stimulation

Video Explanation

https://cdnapisec.kaltura.com/index.php/extwidget/preview/partner_id/2207941/uiconf_id/37292221/entry_id/1_180t7ph3/embed/dynamic

Field Guide for Parkinson's

So far we have taken a look at Parkinson's Disease from a medical viewpoint, analyzing the condition through the hallmark symptoms and presentation. We have discussed the variety of medical and other healthcare professionals who collaborate to provide treatment in a multidimensional fashion to ensure that holistic, patient-centered care is given. The different roles that these providers serve has been mentioned as well as some of the areas that their services are focused on. Finally, some of the main medicinal treatments were mentioned, listing the different classifications of medications, how they work, and why they are used for PD. In the next section, insight will be given into an important component of the healthcare team and a profession that may be misunderstood when it comes to neurologic conditions; physical therapy. A deeper look will be provided into the frameworks for physical therapy for PD as well as the role of PT throughout the course of Parkinson's, and an additional discussion of the specialties that exist within this field when it comes to working with you and others with PD.

Field Guide for Parkinson's

Chapter 3

Physical Therapy

It's only fitting that as a movement disorder, Parkinson's Disease must be addressed with the assistance of professionals that specialize in movement. The importance of all the other team members involved in caring for you cannot be understated, but one key aspect of the team has not yet been mentioned in detail. As described by the American Physical Therapy Association (APTA), physical therapists are these movement experts.[22] The scope of physical therapists (PT) is not limited to rehabilitation of musculoskeletal injuries or post-surgical interventions, but instead spans across a wider dimension. Individuals of all ages with any variety or number of conditions including injuries, disabilities, and other health conditions of an acute or chronic nature which can benefit from physical therapy interventions.[22] They are experts at the nature of movements and all of the components that go into it as well as how the individual's activities or their participation/role in life may be limited as a result of inability to move well.[23] Whether the intervention be restorative to prior ability levels, preventative of injuries or problems that may present in the future as a result of improper or unsafe movements, or compensatory to find ways to move despite limiting circumstances or degenerative diseases, PTs play a critical role in tackling these problems.

When it comes to Parkinson's Disease, physical therapists play a vital role throughout each stage of the condition. Early intervention is important for maximizing the functional ability throughout the progression of the disease but even if this is not achieved, PT intervention is still beneficial even in later stages. In conjunction with pharmacological treatment, physical therapy seeks to reduce the impact and delay the onset of the impairments common to Parkinson's disease. Different learning strategies for gaining or adjusting movement require more research to understand the most effective physical rehabilitation strategy for Parkinson's Disease but based on the pathophysiology of the condition, there are certain approaches or focuses that you might see your physical therapist take that are specific to this condition. When seeking to learn or perfect movement sequences, you might observe that they reduce any "clutter" or external stimuli during the treatment session in order to reduce episodes of freezing during the session.[1] Initially a cue to focus one's attention internally when producing the movement may be applied. Competing sources which demand attention may be removed to further enhance focus through removing anything that might result in dual tasking. Many repetitions are performed in order to engrain the desired movement such that it becomes instinctive and a procedural skill which does not require thinking to perform. Another component of a physical therapy session focusing on practicing specific movements that should be adjusted specifically for Parkinson's disease involves the type practice that is implemented. Whereas a random practice order involves switching between different tasks, back and forth, in a random order, blocked practice involves repeatedly practicing the same task over and over. Blocked practice has been shown to be most effective at improving movement speed and consistency.[24] In desiring to optimize movement techniques and strategies, a physical therapist must choose the proper cueing. Internal cueing is one such type, which involves the individual's understanding of their body and corrections based on such. However, the basal ganglia which is affected in Parkinson's disease, is critical for internal cueing and therefore this process is disrupted. The supplementary motor area of the brain receives input from the basal ganglia to formulate self-initiated movements and generate repetitive, well-learned movements. With the disturbance in this process, other areas of the brain that are involved in movement must be utilized through a different type of cueing. Using both visual and auditory cueing is one such way to bypass the affected brain areas, as these stimuli are processed elsewhere in the central nervous system. Visual cues can include colorful lines on the floor, serving as a target point for walking, or other devices such as a laser light that can be mounted to a cane, walker, or chest harness, and projects a target on the floor serving as a target for walking. Such interventions have evidence supporting their usage to improve both the stride length and velocity of gait.[1,25] The utilization of visual cues continues to evolve with offering of even smaller devices like the image below demonstrates, where the lasers can be attached to individual shoes for those without the requirement of an assistive device. The QR code following the image is a link to a description, detailing how this device works and the impact that they could have.

Field Guide for Parkinson's

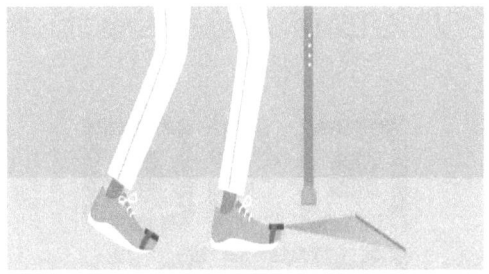

https://parkinsonsdisease.net/news/laser-shoes-gait/

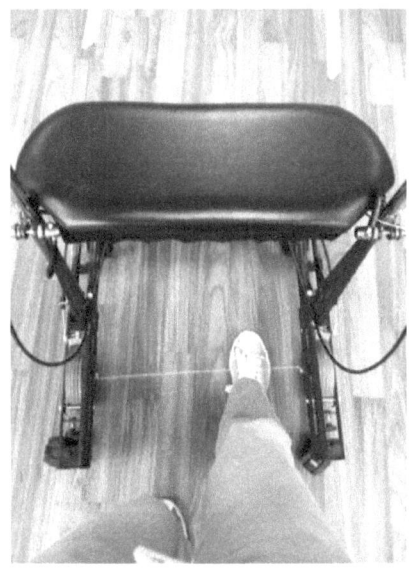

https://www.caregiverproducts.com/assets/images/cis402l-u-step-2-laser-demo.jpg

Field Guide for Parkinson's

RESOURCE ITEM #10: *Laser Shoes Described*

https://parkinsonsdisease.net/news/laser-shoes-gait/

Auditory stimulation is another form of cueing that bypasses the affected pathway in the brain that results in difficulty moving as seen in those with Parkinson's Disease. This could present in the form of simple verbal commands during walking such as saying "big step" or "ready-set-go" but have even more of an impact when delivered rhythmically. Metronomes are a form of rhythmic auditory stimulation (RAS) that has been shown to improve gait speed, cadence, and stride length.[1] An example of metronome use would be taking a step during each beat in order to provide a steady, rhythmic pace of during gait. A growing body of evidence points to the importance of auditory stimulation for improving components of gait, specifically timing and rhythm. The following two QR codes present further information regarding music and auditory stimulation for Parkinson's Disease; the first being a recent study out of The Ohio State University exploring the role of music-based rehabilitation for PD and the second being a short, free book on sound, music and movement in PD.[26]

Both are accessible online through the following links if you have further interest in the subject but resources involving music therapy, specifically through dance can be found in a later chapter. With the evidence reflecting the power of including sound in therapeutic interventions, auditory cueing is critical in successful physical therapy practice for the management of PD. In a subsequent section, more information regarding music therapy can be found.

Field Guide for Parkinson's

RESOURCE ITEM #11: *Music-Based Rehabilitation*

https://www.frontiersin.org/articles/10.3389/fneur.2015.00217/full

RESOURCE ITEM #12: *Sound, Music, and Movement in Parkinson's Disease*

https://www.researchgate.net/profile/Marta_Bienkiewicz/publication/312086115_Sound_Musi c_and_Movement_in_Parkinson%27s_Disease/links/586e7b7508ae6eb871bd9dce/Sound-Music -and-Movement-in-Parkinsons-Disease.pdf

Having established the types of cues preferred for PD specifically, it is time to discuss other interventions that you might perform during a PT session. In addition to the known benefits of exercise on neuroplasticity and counteracting aging both of the body and of the brain, exercise involving high-amplitude movements demonstrate even better improvements in motor performance and in neuroprotection.[1,27,28] The Lee Silverman Voice Treatment (LSVT) Big program, one aspect of the aforementioned LSVT Big & Loud, is based on this concept and has demonstrated significant objective improvements for those who undergo even just 4 weeks of this program. Physical therapists may utilize large, exaggerated movements in their treatment, but to obtain LSVT Big certification one must attend a course which is offered for both physical and occupational therapists (students and assistants included) and covers fundamental treatment principles based on research, key elements of treatment, customization of delivery based on the progression of PD, and more. If you are interested in finding a physical therapist who has LSVT Big certification (or occupational therapist as well), the resource on the following page is a search tool that can locate a clinician with this certification near you.[29]

Field Guide for Parkinson's

RESOURCE ITEM #13: *LSVT BIG Certified Physical Therapists*

https://www.lsvtglobal.com/LSVTFindClinicians

Field Guide for Parkinson's

In addition to exercises focused specifically on movement strategies, physical therapy can include exercises focused on improving flexibility. With rigidity occurring as one of the cardinal features of Parkinson's Disease, interventions directed at improving flexibility and relaxation are necessary for maintaining mobility. Common areas of limitation that may be addressed through flexibility interventions are cervical rotation and retraction, shoulder flexion with trunk extension, trunk rotation, hip/elbow/knee extension, trunk extension, hip abduction, and ankle dorsiflexion. Limitations in these motions could affect bed mobility, gait, and other functional movements and therefore management. Training functional movements such as sit-to-stand, stand-to-sit, bed mobility, gait, and stair negotiation are some of the primary aspects of a physical therapy bout in neurological conditions. These are critical movements in everyday life and are required for successful independent living, and therefore warrant attention and time devoted to improvement. Resistance training is often included in

Field Guide for Parkinson's

Parkinson's Disease management from a physical therapy perspective, specifically following prolonged inactivity, deficits in force production, and poor posture. Weakness can contribute to postural instability, falls, and exertion and resistance training is one way to help prevent these from happening. Furthermore, aside from those with Parkinson's Disease, resistance training has been shown to improve cardiovascular health, improve cognitive abilities, and reducing pain in the general population as well as reducing risk of diabetes, visceral fat, and improving body composition.[30] Balance training is yet another component of a comprehensive physical therapy management program because of the health risk that falling poses and the increased risk of falls that a Parkinson's diagnosis presents.[31] Likewise, a combination of resistance training and balance exercises appears to be a more effective approach at improving a number of outcomes related to muscle activation and balance. Silva-Batista et. al. found that resistance training improved muscle size, activation amount and time, and relaxation time in individuals with Parkinson's compared with a control but that a resistance training with an instability component demonstrated significantly greater improvements than the group that underwent resistance training only, even while undergoing less total training volume.[32] This shows the importance of including both resistance training and instability components in a physical therapy program designed for individuals with Parkinson's Disease and that high amounts of resistance might not be absolutely necessary when an instability component is included as well. Finally, aerobic exercise somewhere in the range of 60% to 80% of the maximum HR is recommended. These programs have been shown to be safe and effective at improving aerobic capacity in individuals with Parkinson's Disease.[1,33,34]

Neurological Clinical Specialists

The Academy of Neurologic Physical Therapy (ANPT) is one of the 18 specialty sections acknowledged within the APTA. Of these 18 specialty sections, it is one of the fastest growing with approximately 6000 members currently.[35] Continuing education programs, conferences, and 8 special interest groups including focuses such as degenerative diseases, spinal cord injuries, assistive technology, balance and falls, etc. are some of the features that this organization offers for physical therapists. The ANPT recognizes the unique challenges and features that present when working with those with Parkinson's or other conditions and seek to offer the best treatment to you through promoting optimal recovery, wellness, and quality of life. Personally, I am of the opinion that it is not required to work with a physical therapist who is a member of the ANPT section of the APTA but as a general rule, the more specific the treatment that you receive is to yourself, and the more versed a therapist is in working with your specific population, the better the outcomes may be. Not only does the Academy of Neurologic Physical Therapy provide a plethora of resources to aid therapists practicing in this field, but they provide information that could be useful for patients. A physical therapist may earn a Neurological Clinical Specialist (NCS) certification through advanced training in the neurological setting and have passed a specialty examination from the American Board of Physical Therapist Specialists.[35]

An initial bout of physical therapy after a Parkinson's diagnosis which focuses on a variety of areas that can be anticipated to need assistance in the future is important in the early management of the disease. Utilizing blocked practice to engrain movement strategies for every area of life including gait, transferring strategies such as going from sitting to standing/supine-to-sit, etc., steps, basically every foreseeable movement in the future with additional help with stepping/ankle/hip reactionary and anticipatory balance strategies because of the increased fall risk and the statistics that are available that indicate the huge impact of falls on mortality. Because new movement patterns are not able to be learned later in the progression of the disorder past a certain point, see a physical therapist as early as possible. If you're already further on in the course of the disease, physical therapy is still important for forming compensatory strategies based on the movement capacity available, maximizing the available functional capacity. Furthermore, physical musculoskeletal impairments can be addressed by physical therapists during these latter stages. After an initial bout of physical therapy, periodic visits can be included to address areas that are challenging or becoming more difficult. LSVT Big certified physical therapists can be beneficial for those with PD especially in the early to mid-stages of Parkinson's disease.

I hope that the preceding chapter has demonstrated the importance of physical therapy in managing Parkinson's Disease. Through the variety of focused interventions, physical therapy covers a widespread area of assistance and expertise especially when it comes to Parkinson's disease. Undoubtedly, there will be certain aspects of physical therapy that have not been discussed given the broad nature of the field but the aforementioned techniques are just some things that you may perform at a physical therapy session or that you wish to discuss with your physical therapist as well as some of the alternative/adjunctive therapeutic methods and modalities that will be discussed shortly, some of which may even be offered by certain physical therapists, such as dry needling.

Despite the beneficial aspects of physical therapy and all of the other interventions that are offered through the multidisciplinary care team, there needs to be additional help. You won't be able to (or want to) see a physical therapist or medical professional every day for the rest of your life so other strategies should be explored and implemented. In this next section, alternative interventions and resources will be offered. These are only here as a description of them and not as advice whether to try them or not. Examine these at your own discretion and use the resource items to follow simply as ideas and as a way to say that the options are endless; that there are groups and resources that you might already partake in to some degree that can be catered and adjusted for someone living with Parkinson's disease. To conclude the chapter, the following QR code is included as a resource for finding a physical therapist near you with search criteria including the option to search specifically for a NCS certified physical therapist.

Field Guide for Parkinson's

RESOURCE ITEM #14: *Find a PT*

https://aptaapps.apta.org/APTAPTDirectory/FindAPTDirectory.aspx

Field Guide for Parkinson's

Chapter 4

Alternative and Adjunctive Methods

Dry needling

Acupuncture and dry needling have been exploratory methods utilized to aid in treatment of symptoms of PD. Pain relief and relaxing muscles and reducing fatigue through targeted dry needling, acupuncture or electroacupuncture has been shown in some cases to be beneficial. Rather than having to seek out a specific acupuncturist, physical therapists who have certifications in dry needling can be utilized to minimize the need for adding yet another provider into your health care team. Physical Therapists can obtain a level I or level II certification with level I focused on the periphery, soft tissue, and ligaments whereas level II focuses on the spine and more central regions.[36] The following two resources included are an explanation of dry needling and a resource for finding a physical therapist including those with specialties.

Field Guide for Parkinson's

RESOURCE ITEM #15: *Dry Needling Explained*

https://www.mayoclinichealthsystem.org/hometown-health/speaking-of-health/on-pins-and-needles-just-what-is-dry-needling

Music Therapy

The importance of auditory cueing has already been discussed in addition to the inclusion of two resources: the article on music therapy on Parkinson's and the book about music and sound therapy for Parkinson's.[26] Music therapy is helpful in reducing freezing, improving gait and speech, increasing postural control, and improving cognition according to one study.[37] Not only is this a potentially effective component in the management of Parkinson's Disease, but it can be a fun way to socialize with other individuals dealing with the same condition.[37] The following QR link provides access to the American Music Therapy Association where more information can be found with an additional QR code following the first, which leads to a search tool for finding a music therapist.

Field Guide for Parkinson's

RESOURCE ITEM #16: *American Music Therapy Association*

https://www.musictherapy.org/

Field Guide for Parkinson's

***RESOURCE ITEM #17:** Find a Music Therapist*

https://netforum.avectra.com/eweb/DynamicPage.aspx?Site=amta2&WebCode=IndSearch

Boxing

Rock Steady Boxing is a non-profit organization of increasing popularity that aims to improve the quality of life of individuals with Parkinson's Disease through a non-contact boxing based fitness curriculum. Boxing drills and conditioning with emphasis on agility, speed, endurance, accuracy, hand-eye coordination, footwork and strength are implemented with varying intensity based on ability.[36,38] Rock Steady may be a good program to look into to increase physical fitness, although critics of this program state that despite its growing popularity, the benefits of Rock Steady have limited evidence.[39] Similarly, the risks and safety guidelines have not been demonstrated. Could it be simply that individuals in these classes are reaping the benefits of regular exercise rather than a magical benefit that is specific to boxing? The benefits of regular, high-intensity exercise have already been spelled out in a previous chapter and the evidence is not difficult to find with a simple search. So could it be that finding a form of exercise that is enjoyable and can be adhered to consistently is the key, instead of something specific to boxing? As with any of these adjunctive and alternative therapies, this goes under the "use your judgment" category. The following QR code as found on the following page leads to a search tool for finding a Rock Steady Boxing class close to you.

Field Guide for Parkinson's

RESOURCE ITEM #18: *Rock Steady Boxing*

https://www.rocksteadyboxing.org/find-a-class/

Pilates

You may have previously heard claims that Pilates is a very effective form of exercise for those with Parkinson's disease because of its popularity. With the goal of Pilates being to improve postural alignment, core strength, and balance, it is very possible that you might benefit from this.[36] Additionally, the group exercise setting is a great way to improve social ties and maintain adherence to exercise. Improvements in cognition are also claimed to be a benefit of Pilates, which is reasonable given the known neuroprotective and cognitive benefits from partaking in regular exercise. However, research efforts to critically examine benefits specific to Parkinson's patients in comparison to other forms of exercise is sparse. Whereas there are some studies looking at the effects of Pilates on Parkinson's Disease, the quality of these studies is poor with many only including single-subject trials which may not be generalizable to the larger population.[40] Similar to Rock Steady Boxing, could the benefits simply be due to

Field Guide for Parkinson's

sustained adherence to an exercise program rather than a specific component of Pilates. If this is true, even though there may be no direct improvements from Pilates that can't be offered by other types of exercise, if Pilates is something that interests you and that you feel that you could commit to regularly attending, it could be a viable option and something to look into. A search tool for pilates classes near you can be found through the QR code on the next page, although take note that these classes are not specific to individuals with Parkinson's and should be considered when signing up for a class. An instructor that is familiar working with individuals with Parkinson's may be important in order to fully appreciate the potential benefits of Pilates. Some physical therapists may have experience with Pilates or implementing Pilates-esque methods during rehabilitation sessions. Resource item #20 provides information on how Pilates may be implemented for physical rehabilitation.

Field Guide for Parkinson's

RESOURCE ITEM #19: Pilates Studio Finder

https://www.pilates.com/community/studio-finder

Field Guide for Parkinson's

RESOURCE ITEM #20: *Pilates for Rehabilitation*

https://sites.pilates.com/rehab/

Reiki

Reiki is based on the concept that we have a "life force energy" that flows through us and that having a low life force can cause illness and stress whereas a high life force can cause greater health and happiness. Strange? Perhaps, but there are testimonials that praise the benefits of Reiki reduction in tremors and rigidity. It is true that stress and anxiety can result in increased intensity of tremors and the relaxing and calming nature of Reiki could be a beneficial practice. For those who find the concept of Reiki odd, see the section on Mindfulness, Ayurveda, or the Feldenkrais method for methods to improve the mind-body relationship.[36,41] Testimonials on Reiki for Parkinson's can be found through the resource item on the next page. Subsequently, a link to a class locator can be found through Resource Item #22.

Field Guide for Parkinson's

RESOURCE ITEM #21: _Reiki Testimonials_

https://reikiforwellness.org/reiki-%26-parkinsons

Field Guide for Parkinson's

RESOURCE ITEM #22: *Reiki Locator*

https://iarp.org/find-reiki-practitioner-teacher/

Field Guide for Parkinson's

<u>Qigong</u>

Taking a short flight over the Sea of Japan to China, the practice of Qigong has similar claims of healing and relieving symptoms of Parkinson's Disease. Like Reiki, Qigong focuses on the flow of energy and in connecting the mental and physical health through posture, movement, breathing, self-massage, sound, and focus.[42] There is some evidence that supports the practice of Qigong in reducing motor symptoms of Parkinson's as well as mental state through a decrease in depressive symptoms.[43,44] See the following resource item, accessible through the QR code or the link at the bottom of the next page for an informational video about the fundamentals of Qigong as described by the National Qigong Association. Resource item #24 is a search tool that can be used to find a Qigong teacher near you.

Field Guide for Parkinson's

RESOURCE ITEM #23: *Discovering Qigong*

https://www.nqa.org/what-is-qigong-

Field Guide for Parkinson's

RESOURCE ITEM #24: *Find a Qigong Teacher*

https://www.nqa.org/find-a-teacher#/

Tai Chi

Yet another practice that seeks to connect the mind and body through movement, focused attention, and motor activities incorporating balance, coordination, and flexibility, Tai Chi has shown potential for slowing the disease progression and improving function.[36,45] It may also be beneficial in increasing stride length, functional reach and lowering fall risk.[46] The amount of Tai Chi courses, instructors, and programs is vast and difficult to put in one succinct location but the next resource item is a search tool for locating Tai Chi and/or Qigong classes. With any program aimed at improving balance, finding a safe location or supervision is recommended in order to reduce any risk of falling, especially if you have any fear or uneasiness when it comes to balance and fall-risk. Resource item #26 is a brief example of what a Tai Chi session might look like to serve not as a recommended practice but rather as a small sample of what could be expected.

Field Guide for Parkinson's

RESOURCE ITEM #25: *Tai Chi or Qigong class/teacher locator*

http://www.americantaichi.net/TaiChiQigongClass.asp

Field Guide for Parkinson's

RESOURCE ITEM #26: *Tai Chi video example*

https://www.youtube.com/watch?v=ZxcNBejxlzs

Field Guide for Parkinson's

Ayurveda

Ayurveda also taps into this "mind-body connection" in its concept of taking actions along a path that is suitable to the mind-body type that each person has. Ayurveda is one of the oldest systems of natural healing that evaluates every aspect of wellbeing through determining whether or not it is an appropriate measure based on one's mind-body type.[47,48] Herbal medications are one component of Ayurveda including the Mucuna pruriens plant which will be discussed next. Access the QR code on the next page for information regarding Ayurveda.

RESOURCE ITEM #27: *Ayurveda Explained*

https://www.epda.eu.com/living-well/therapies/complementary-therapies/ayurveda/

Mucuna pruriens

The mucuna seed is a commonly used herb used in Ayurvedic treatment which contains the precursor to dopamine, levodopa, the substance used in the medication l-dopa. Side-stepping the artificial manufacturing of levodopa, mucuna is a way to access it in a natural form with few side effects.[36] One study even claims that the mucuna seed powder can possess some advantages over manufactured levodopa with respect to long-term treatment of PD.[49] In a previous chapter, the limited usable period of l-dopa was spelled out. This is not an alternative to prescribed medications but could be something to look into and discuss with your care team. The QR code on the next page leads to more information about the Mucuna pruriens plant from the American Parkinson Disease Association.

Field Guide for Parkinson's

RESOURCE ITEM #28: *Mucuna Pruriens*

https://www.apdaparkinson.org/article/mucuna-pruriens-for-parkinsons-disease/

Field Guide for Parkinson's

Mindfulness

If you aren't quite comfortable committing to something like Ayurveda, Qigong, or Reiki, mindfulness could be a way to practice awareness and meditation in a way that you may find to be less "out there" or uncomfortable. Mindfulness practice has recognized benefits of stress reduction, improved concentration and mood, improving sleep, reducing the effects of aging and pain, and more.[36] Specific to Parkinson's Disease, one study reported that structural changes in the brain such as increased density within basal ganglia and throughout various other regions of the brain.[50] As a well-accepted means of improving one's awareness, reducing stress/anxiety and all of the other previously mentioned benefits, this practice is one that could be recommended for anyone with the additional benefits specifically shown in those with Parkinson's Disease serving as an additional endorsement. The first of the multiple resource items offered for mindfulness is a link to 10 popular guided meditations with a variety of focuses. Secondly, two video resources are provided, the first of which gives a brief general perspective on mindfulness and the second offering another explanation of mindfulness as well as several steps for beginning mindfulness meditation. Finally, the last QR code for this section on mindfulness leads to a number of guided mindfulness videos from the Parkinson's Foundation, as a part of their Mindfulness Mondays series.

Field Guide for Parkinson's

RESOURCE ITEM #29: *10 Guided Meditations*

https://www.mindful.org/mindfuls-top-10-guided-meditations-of-2018/

Field Guide for Parkinson's

RESOURCE ITEM #30: *Mindfulness Animation*

https://www.youtube.com/watch?v=w6T02g5hnT4

Field Guide for Parkinson's

RESOURCE ITEM #31: *Mindfulness Explanation*

https://www.youtube.com/watch?v=mjtfyuTTQFY

Field Guide for Parkinson's

RESOURCE ITEM #32: *Mindfulness Mondays*

https://www.parkinson.org/Living-with-Parkinsons/Resources-and-Support/PD-Health-at-Home/Mindfulness-Mondays

Yoga

Yoga therapy is a form of yoga designed to help individuals get relief from symptoms of a multitude of conditions. Yoga therapists have undergone specialized training for these conditions including Parkinson's Disease and may offer classes on an individual or group basis.[36] Evidence indicates that yoga may be beneficial in improving steadiness of gait, reducing tremors, flexibility, strength, posture, and overall well-being.[51,52] The first of two resource items regarding yoga is a link to yoga positions beneficial to individuals with Parkinson's as provided by Yoga International. These should be discussed with your health care team prior to jumping in and beginning these on your own. A certified yoga therapist should be consulted for safe application of a yoga therapy program and in sight of this, the second resource item for this section is a search tool for locating a certified yoga therapist near you.

Field Guide for Parkinson's

RESOURCE ITEM #33: *Yoga International Recommended Positions*

https://yogainternational.com/article/view/yoga-therapy-and-parkinsons-disease

Field Guide for Parkinson's

RESOURCE ITEM #34: *Yoga Therapist Locator*

https://www.iayt.org/search/custom.asp?id=4160

Dancing

Dancing has demonstrated improvements in individuals with Parkinson's Disease on a number of physical therapy outcome measures such as the Berg Balance Scale, six minute walk test, and stride length which correlate with a number of different outcomes. The Tango is one style of dance with more improvements in deficits associated with Parkinson's although other dances such as the Waltz and Foxtrot can benefit balance and movement as well.[53] Dance classes catered for those with Parkinson's Disease are offered with instructors trained in dance therapy and can be found using the search tool offered in the following resource item.

Field Guide for Parkinson's

RESOURCE ITEM #35: *Dance Therapy Locator*

https://danceforparkinsons.org/find-a-class/class-locations/united-states

Art Therapy

Art therapy may not have the data that some of these other complementary therapies do but it could be an additional avenue to explore for those interested in artistic endeavours of any kind. The American Art Therapy Association claims benefits of art therapy such as reduced anxiety, improved social ties, and mental health management. Perhaps practicing fine motor skills such as handling an art brush could serve as another component of art therapy that could be meaningful in the management of PD.[54] The benefits of this kind of therapy are not well discussed in relation to Parkinson's Disease in particular but because of the general benefits that are offered through art therapy, this could something worth exploring.[36] The American Art Therapy Association offers an Art Therapist Locator which can be accessed through the following QR code.

Field Guide for Parkinson's

RESOURCE ITEM #36: *Art Therapy Locator*

https://arttherapy.org/art-therapist-locator/

Massage Therapy

If you've ever had a massage, you can vouch for the relaxed state that you feel afterwards. Naturally this would be a beneficial modality for those with Parkinson's Disease given the rigid state that can exist through the overactive musculature of opposing muscle groups. Little risk is associated with massage therapy and there are a multitude of locations where these services are offered.[36] The American Massage Therapy Association even offers a search tool for locating a massage therapist near your location which can be found on the next page.

Field Guide for Parkinson's

RESOURCE ITEM #37: _Massage Therapist Locator_

https://www.amtamassage.org/find-massage-therapist/

Cannabinoids

Evolving research exists in relation to cannabinoids as a therapeutic modality with further evidence coming in as more and more states push for legalization. Studies like one conducted by Kluger et al. examining the potential for cannabinoids as a therapeutic technique continue to be performed although too much is still unknown in terms of risks associated versus potential benefits to allow for this to be recommended as an approach worth exploring.[36,55]

Feldenkrais Method

    Finally, the last alternative/adjunct therapy that will be presented in this chapter is the Feldenkrais Method. In a similar light to the concepts that have been presented through various other methods in this chapter, the Feldenkrais method is centered around the mind-body relationship and that in order to change movement, we must change our mind. The benefits cited include better balance, breathing, coordination, flexibility, etc. It can be taught in a group or individual setting with instruction focused on teaching movement sequences. Included on the following page is a resource further describing the Feldenkrais Method followed by a resource for finding classes near you.[36]

Field Guide for Parkinson's

RESOURCE ITEM #38: _Feldenkrais Method Described_

https://feldenkrais.com/

Field Guide for Parkinson's

RESOURCE ITEM #39: *Feldenkrais Locator*

https://feldenkrais.com/location-search/

Chapter 5

Fall Prevention Programs (outside of PT)

Field Guide for Parkinson's

Falls play a massive role in disrupting the health and life of older individuals and those with Parkinson's Disease. In older adults, they are the leading cause of emergency department visits, hospital admissions, and unintentional death and even falling once doubles the risk of a second fall. Traumatic brain injuries most commonly occur from falls, nearly all hip fractures are caused by falls (95%), and 20% of falls result in a head injury or fracture.[31] For those with Parkinson's fall risk is even further increased. With this in mind, interventions aimed at reducing the risk of falling should be a large area of focus. Physical therapy is one way that this is addressed, but in this chapter a number of additional prevention programs are discussed. Each of these programs are listed and described by the National Council on Aging and can be found at the QR code on the following page but will also be listed individually in this chapter.

Field Guide for Parkinson's

RESOURCE ITEM #40: <u>NCOA Falls Prevention</u>

https://www.ncoa.org/healthy-aging/falls-prevention/falls-prevention-programs-for-older-adults-2/

Field Guide for Parkinson's

A Matter of Balance

This program includes 8, two-hour sessions over the course of 8 weeks designed to reduce the risk of falling and increasing activity levels. A structured group intervention teaches ways to reduce the fear of falling, minimize risk factors in the home and community that could lead to falls, and improve strength and balance. This is not limited to those with PD but also for individuals who are concerned about falling, have fallen in the past, or are seeking to improve flexibility, balance, and strength. For this reason, A Matter of Balance could be a good intervention for those who would like additional assistance with balance outside of physical therapy or if you would like to be able to go through this program with a significant other, friend, or acquaintance who also wishes to prevent falls. This program has the benefit of working in groups, so you are able to have other individuals there going through this course with you rather than having only the individualized care from a PT. Once again, this is not a substitute for the patient-specific interventions that can be offered by a PT but might be a nice resource to utilize in adjunct.[36,56] *The following QR code leads to a document of contact information for locations offering this program.*

Field Guide for Parkinson's

RESERVE ITEM #41: *A Matter of Balance*

Contacts

https://www.mainehealth.org/-/media/Elder-Services/Matter-of-Balance/Files/MOB-MT-Contact-Info-010820.xlsx

Bingocize

Bingocize includes 2 one-hour sessions over the course of 10 weeks where participants play a bingo-like game combined with exercise and health education. Upper body strength, lower body strength, health knowledge on fall risk, and walking speed were all shown to increase following a study observing the effects of this course.[57,58] A mobile application is offered in addition to a print-out sheet of the program. This is a relatively new intervention and thus the implementation is not widespread and readily available. The application itself costs $250 and is unavailable on the Google or Apple app store currently. At the present time this might not be the most viable option but may be something to keep an eye out for in the future. Similar to the Rock-Steady Boxing program, the benefits of Bingocize may not be exclusive to this program in particular. Instead, being more active, moving more, and exercising with moderate to vigorous intensity have been established as an effective means of improving health and wellbeing regardless of how they *are implemented. If Bingocize sounds like a format of exercise that you'd be interested in, perhaps it would be something to consider looking into but if not, there are other ways to get the benefits of exercise other than Bingocize.*

Field Guide for Parkinson's

RESOURCE ITEM #42: *Bingocize Information*

https://www.wku.edu/bingocize/

Enhance Fitness

This program is a low-cost group exercise program with a focus on both physical activity and fall prevention. One hour sessions are held 3 times per week with each including a regimen designed to impact cardiovascular health, balance, strength, and stretching. This is another non-Parkinson's specific program that seeks to improve overall physical health in a group format that could be something to consider exploring as a way to get the recommended physical activity amounts with the additional benefits of improving balance. Again, physical therapists are the movement experts and are the go-to resource for identifying factors that are specific to the individual in regards to fall-risk in and overall movement but this could be an additional way to further reduce risk of falling and improving health with the perks of being in a group environment.[56] The following QR code is a link to a site locator for the Enhance programs offered across the country.

RESOURCE ITEM #43: *Enhance Fitness Site Locator*

https://projectenhance.org/locations/

Otago Exercise Program

When searching for a physical therapist, we have previously mentioned the LSVT Big certification that some therapists may have and which could be beneficial, however, not necessarily required. One other training that you might search for when looking for a physical therapist, is the Otago Exercise Program. This program which is implemented by the physical therapist as a part of their interventions is composed of 17 specific strength and balance exercises targeting fall reduction. It consists of an 8-week series of physical therapy appointments followed by a self-management phase for 4-10 months. The program claims to have a 35-40% reduction in falls for their older adult patients who receive this treatment.[36,59] The following QR code leads to a listing of physical therapists who have received training in the Otago Exercise Program.

Field Guide for Parkinson's

RESOURCE ITEM #44: *Otago Therapists Listings*

https://woodland.med.unc.edu/CGECPT/CGECPT/CGECPT

YMCA Moving for Better Balance

This is a 12 week program led by an instructor with focuses on improving strength, mobility, flexibility, and balance in order to increase overall health and functioning. It is based on eight movements modified in order to aid in fall prevention which are introduced through the principles of Tai Chi. YMCAs across the country offer this service which does not require a YMCA membership. The QR code on the next page is a link to a YMCA locator to find one near you if this sounds like an option you'd like to explore.[36]

Field Guide for Parkinson's

RESOURCE ITEM #45: YMCA locations

https://www.ymca.net/find-your-y/

Chapter 6

PD Staples and Conclusion

Field Guide for Parkinson's

The final two resources that will be presented can be utilized for a variety of questions related to Parkinson's Disease. These offer assistance and information about finding groups, exercise opportunities, current research about Parkinson's and more. Rather than separate these final resources by a descriptor preceding their QR code, a brief overview of all of them will be given first. The first is the American Parkinson Disease Association. This organization was founded in 1961 and has spent the years since providing education, awareness, support and research on the topic of Parkinson's. Next is the Parkinson's Foundation which seeks to help improve the quality of life for those with PD through improving care and advancing research towards curing this disease.

Field Guide for Parkinson's

RESOURCE ITEM #46: *American Parkinson's Disease Association Website*

1-800-223-2732

https://www.apdaparkinson.org/

Field Guide for Parkinson's

RESOURCE ITEM #47: *Parkinson's Foundation*

Helpline: 1-800-473-4636

Email: helpline@parkinson.org

https://www.parkinson.org/

Field Guide for Parkinson's

To conclude this exploration of Parkinson's Disease from its etiology, medicinal and medical management, as well as alternative methods, I want to begin by reiterating that this book is NOT a recommendation for the management of PD but only serves to reveal the different areas of practice and exploratory methods that are being researched or looked into. These alternative methods are not a replacement for the treatment that healthcare professionals provide but could be items of discussion with your medical team. Physical therapy is a key aspect of this team throughout life and has functional benefits for those across the various stages of the disease. Research on Parkinson's Disease is ever evolving and new therapeutic techniques are presented every year so fortunately by the time you are reading this book, there is likely a novel technique being examined that has been bypassed at the time of this book's composition. As you know, being diagnosed with Parkinson's is a difficult thing to grapple with. My hope is that through these resources, you can feel encouraged by the extensive amount of assistance out there. With the descriptions of the alternative adjunctive therapies you may have noticed a theme emerging. Emphasis on the interaction between mental and physical wellness was addressed in nearly every one of these resources with repeated attention given to promoting exercise, social interaction, and mindfulness. These components are not unique to Parkinson's Disease but, instead, are items that everyone should attend to. Regardless of where you are in life, there is the possibility to make improvements in these areas and improve one's quality of life, for one's overall well being is not subject to a diagnosis but to the care that they give themselves in relation to these components.

Field Guide for Parkinson's

Resource Guide

Consolidated Index

Field Guide for Parkinson's

RESOURCE ITEM #1: PD Explained	12
RESOURCE ITEM #2: Neurologist Database	17
RESOURCE ITEM #3: MDS Database	19
RESOURCE ITEM #4 LSVT Explained	24
RESOURCE ITEM #5: Dietician Search	26
RESOURCE ITEM #6: Neuropsychologist Directory	29
RESOURCE ITEM #7: Medication Form	36
RESOURCE ITEM #8: Aware in Care Kit	37
RESOURCE ITEM #9: Deep Brain Stimulation Video Explanation	46
RESOURCE ITEM #10: Laser Shoes Described	56
RESOURCE ITEM #11 Music-Based Rehabilitation	59
RESOURCE ITEM #12: Sound, Music & Movement in PD	60
RESOURCE ITEM #13: LSVT BIG Certified Physical Therapists	63
RESOURCE ITEM #14: Find a PT	72
RESOURCE ITEM #15: Dry Needling Explained	75
RESOURCE ITEM #16: American Music Therapy Association	77
RESOURCE ITEM #17: Find a Music Therapist	78

Field Guide for Parkinson's

RESOURCE ITEM #18: Rock Steady Boxing	81
RESOURCE ITEM #19: Pilates Studio Finder	84
RESOURCE ITEM #20: Pilates for Rehabilitation	85
RESOURCE ITEM #21: Reiki Testimonials	87
RESOURCE ITEM #22: Reiki Locator	88
RESOURCE ITEM #23: Discovering Qigong	90
RESOURCE ITEM #24: Find a Qigong Teacher	91
RESOURCE ITEM #25: Tai Chi/Qigong Class/Teacher Locator	93
RESOURCE ITEM #26: Tai Chi Video Example	94
RESOURCE ITEM #27: Ayurveda Explained	96
RESOURCE ITEM #28: Mucuna Pruriens	98
RESOURCE ITEM #29: 10 Guided Meditations	101
RESOURCE ITEM #30: Mindfulness Animation	102
RESOURCE ITEM #31: Mindfulness Explanation	103
RESOURCE ITEM #32: Mindfulness Mondays	104
RESOURCE ITEM #33: Yoga International Recommended Positions	106
RESOURCE ITEM #34: Yoga Therapist Locator	107

Field Guide for Parkinson's

RESOURCE ITEM #35: Dance Therapy Locator	109
RESOURCE ITEM #36: Art Therapy Locator	111
RESOURCE ITEM #37: Massage Therapist Locator	113
RESOURCE ITEM #38: Feldenkrais Method Described	116
RESOURCE ITEM #39: Feldenkrais Locator	117
RESOURCE ITEM #40: NCOA Falls Prevention	120
RESOURCE ITEM #41: A Matter of Balance Contacts	123
RESOURCE ITEM #42: Bingocize Information	126
RESOURCE ITEM #43: Enhance Fitness Site Locator	128
RESOURCE ITEM #44: Otago Therapists Listings	130
RESOURCE ITEM #45: YMCA Locations	132
RESOURCE ITEM #46: American Parkinson's Disease Association Website	135
RESOURCE ITEM #47: Parkinson's Foundation	136

Field Guide for Parkinson's

References

1. O'Sullivan, S., Schmitz, T. and Fulk, G., 2019. *Physical Rehabilitation*. Philadelphia, Pa: F.A. Davis.

2. Alexander GE. Biology of Parkinson's disease: pathogenesis and pathophysiology of a multisystem neurodegenerative disorder. *Dialogues Clin Neurosci*. 2004;6(3):259-280.

3. Triarhou LC. Dopamine and Parkinson's Disease. In: *Madame Curie Bioscience Database* [Internet]. Austin (TX): Landes Bioscience; 2000-2013. Available from: https://www.ncbi.nlm.nih.gov/books/NBK6271/

4. Chen JY, Wang EA, Cepeda C, Levine MS. Dopamine imbalance in Huntington's disease: a mechanism for the lack of behavioral flexibility. *Front Neurosci*. 2013;7:114. Published 2013 Jul 4. doi:10.3389/fnins.2013.00114

5. Postuma RB, Berg D, Stern M, Poewe W, Olanow CW, Oertel W, Obeso J, Marek K, Litvan I, Lang AE, Halliday G, Goetz CG, Gasser T, Dubois B, Chan P, Bloem BR, Adler CH, Deuschl G. MDS

clinical diagnostic criteria for Parkinson's disease. Mov Disord. 2015 Oct;30(12):1591-601. doi: 10.1002/mds.26424. PMID: 26474316.

6. Building a Parkinson's Care Team | Everyday Health. EverydayHealth.com. Accessed October 21, 2020. https://www.everydayhealth.com/hs/parkinsons-caregiver-guide/care-team/

7. Becoming a Physical Therapist. APTA. https://www.apta.org/your-career/careers-in-physical-therapy/becoming-a-pt#:~:text=Physical%20therapists%20are%20movement%20experts

8. International Parkinson and Movement Disorder Society. mds.movementdisorders.org. Accessed October 21, 2020. https://mds.movementdisorders.org/directory/

9. Movement Disorder Specialists. The Michael J. Fox Foundation for Parkinson's Research | Parkinson's Disease. Published 2019. https://www.michaeljfox.org/news/movement-disorder-specialists

10. Howley EK. Are PAs Part of the Solution to the Physician Shortage? US News & World Report. Published 2018. https://health.usnews.com/health-care/patient-advice/articles/2018-12-24/are-pas-part-of-the-solution-to-the-physician-shortage

11. NT Contributor. How to care for people with Parkinson's disease | Nursing Times. Nursing Times. Published April 13, 2012. https://www.nursingtimes.net/clinical-archive/neurology/how-to-care-for-people-with-parkinsons-disease-13-04-2012/

12. Chapman M. Parkinson's Foundation Opens Fellowship Program for Nurses Seeking Specialty. Accessed October 21, 2020. https://parkinsonsnewstoday.com/2020/01/24/parkinsons-foundation-opens-nurse-fellowship-program/#:~:text=The%20Parkinson

13. Welsby E, Berrigan S, Laver K. Effectiveness of occupational therapy intervention for people with Parkinson's disease: Systematic review. Aust Occup Ther J. 2019 Dec;66(6):731-738. doi: 10.1111/1440-1630.12615. Epub 2019 Oct 10. PMID: 31599467.

14. Isaacson S, O'Brien A, Lazaro JD, Ray A, Fluet G. The JFK BIG study: the impact of LSVT BIG® on dual task walking and mobility in persons with Parkinson's disease. J Phys Ther Sci. 2018;30(4):636-641. doi:10.1589/jpts.30.636

15. LSVT Big & Loud. Davis Phinney Foundation. Accessed October 21, 2020. https://davisphinneyfoundation.org/lsvt-big-loud/

16. What is LSVT LOUD. Lsvtglobal.com. Published 2015. Accessed October 21, 2020. https://www.lsvtglobal.com/LSVTLoud#bestTimeToStartSection

17. Wahass SH. The role of psychologists in health care delivery. J Family Community Med. 2005;12(2):63-70.

18. Becoming Certified – ABCN. theabcn.org. Accessed October 21, 2020. https://theabcn.org/becoming-certified/

19. Parkinson's Disease Foundation: Medications and Treatments. Retreieved April 23, 2012, fromwww.pdf.org/en/meds_treatments.

20. Deep Brain Stimulation for Parkinson's Disease | Cleveland Clinic. Cleveland Clinic. Published 2019.

https://my.clevelandclinic.org/health/treatments/4080-deep-brain-stimulation-for-parkinsons-disease-patients

21. Ferrucci, R., Bocci, T., Cortese, F. et al. Cerebellar transcranial direct current stimulation in neurological disease. cerebellum ataxias 3, 16 (2016). https://doi.org/10.1186/s40673-016-0054-2

22. Becoming a Physical Therapist. APTA. https://www.apta.org/your-career/careers-in-physical-therapy/becoming-a-pt

23. The International Classification of Functioning, Disability, and Health: Overview (No CEUs). learningcenter.apta.org. Accessed October 21, 2020. https://learningcenter.apta.org/Student/MyCourse.aspx?id=ada8ed39-d7be-4629-9a0a-f55d41e05b04&ProgramID=dcca7f06-4cd9-4530-b9d3-4ef7d2717b5d

24. Behrman, A, Cauraugh, J, and Light, K: Practice as an intervention to improve speeded motor performance and motor learning in Parkinson's disease. A systematic review. Clin Rehabil 19:695, 2005.

25. Lewis, G, Byblow, W, and Walt, S: Stride length regulation in Parkinson's disease: The use of extrinsic visual cues. Brain 123:2077, 2000.

26. Schiavio, A. and Altenmüller, E., 2020. Exploring Music-Based Rehabilitation For Parkinsonism Through Embodied Cognitive Science.

27. Vecchio LM, Meng Y, Xhima K, Lipsman N, Hamani C, Aubert I. The Neuroprotective Effects of Exercise: Maintaining a Healthy Brain Throughout Aging. Brain Plast. 2018;4(1):17-52. Published 2018 Dec 12. doi:10.3233/BPL-180069

28. Hötting K, Röder B. Beneficial effects of physical exercise on neuroplasticity and cognition. Neuroscience and biobehavioral reviews. 2013;37(9 Pt B):2243-2257. doi:10.1016/j.neubiorev.2013.04.005

29. Get LSVT BIG Certified. Lsvtglobal.com. Published 2020. Accessed October 21, 2020. https://www.lsvtglobal.com/Get_LSVTBig_Certified

30. Westcott WL. Resistance training is medicine: effects of strength training on health. Curr Sports Med Rep. 2012

Jul-Aug;11(4):209-16. doi: 10.1249/JSR.0b013e31825dabb8. PMID: 22777332.

31. Falls Prevention Facts. NCOA. Published June 4, 2018. https://www.ncoa.org/news/resources-for-reporters/get-the-facts/falls-prevention-facts/

32. Silva-Batista C, Corcos DM, Barroso R. Instability training improves neuromuscular outcome in Parkinson's Disease. Medicine & Science in Sports & Exercise 2017; 49(4): 652-660.

33. Bergen, J, et. al: Aerobic exercise intervention improves aerobic capacity and movement initiation in Parkinson's disease patients. NeuroRehabilitation 17:161, 2002.

34. Schenkman, M, et. al: Endurance training to improve economy of movement of people with Parkinson disease: Three case reports. Phys Ther 88:63, 2008.

35. Find a Neurologic Physical Therapist. www.neuropt.org. https://www.neuropt.org/consumer-info/what-is-a-neurologic-physical-therapist

36. A Resource Guide of 19 Complementary Therapies for People with Parkinson's. Davis Phinney Foundation. Accessed

October 21, 2020. https://davisphinneyfoundation.org/a-resource-guide-of-19-complementary-therapies-for-people-with-parkinsons/

37. Raglio A. Music Therapy Interventions in Parkinson's Disease: The State-of-the-Art. Front Neurol. 2015;6:185. Published 2015 Aug 31. doi:10.3389/fneur.2015.00185

38. Rock Steady About. www.rocksteadyboxing.org. Accessed October 21, 2020. https://www.rocksteadyboxing.org/about/

39. Morris, M., Ellis, T., Jazayeri, D., Heng, H., Thomson, A., Balasundaram, A. and Slade, S., 2020. Boxing For Parkinson's Disease: Has Implementation Accelerated Beyond Current Evidence?.

40. Suárez-Iglesias D, Miller KJ, Seijo-Martínez M, Ayán C. Benefits of Pilates in Parkinson's Disease: A Systematic Review and Meta-Analysis. Medicina (Kaunas). 2019;55(8):476. Published 2019 Aug 13. doi:10.3390/medicina55080476

41. Association EPD. Reiki. www.epda.eu.com. Accessed October 21, 2020. https://www.epda.eu.com/living-well/therapies/complementar

y-therapies/reiki/#:~:text=Some%20of%20the%20potential%20 benefits%20in%20Parkinson%E2%80%99s%20cited

42. What is Qigong? www.nqa.org. https://www.nqa.org/what-is-qigong-

43. Schmitz-Hübsch T, Pyfer D, Kielwein K, Fimmers R, Klockgether T, Wüllner U. Qigong exercise for the symptoms of Parkinson's disease: a randomized, controlled pilot study. Mov Disord. 2006 Apr;21(4):543-8. doi: 10.1002/mds.20705. PMID: 16229022.

44. Liu XL, Chen S, Wang Y. Effects of Health Qigong Exercises on Relieving Symptoms of Parkinson's Disease. Evid Based Complement Alternat Med. 2016;2016:5935782. doi:10.1155/2016/5935782

45. Li Q, Liu J, Dai f, et al. Tai Chi versus routine exercise in patients with early- or mild-stage Parkinson's disease: a retrospective cohort analysis [published online February 10, 2020]. Braz J Med Biol Res. doi: 10.1590/1414-431x20199171.

46. Li F, Harmer P, Fitzgerald K, et al. Tai chi and postural stability in patients with Parkinson's disease. N Engl J Med. 2012;366(6):511-519. doi:10.1056/NEJMoa1107911

47. The Key to Perfect Health. Chopra. Published March 14, 2013. Accessed October 21, 2020. https://chopra.com/articles/the-key-to-perfect-health?_ga=2.201768085.507446227.1533316228-1359001834.1533316228

48. Association EPD. Ayurveda. www.epda.eu.com. Accessed October 21, 2020. https://www.epda.eu.com/living-well/therapies/complementary-therapies/ayurveda/

49. Katzenschlager R, Evans A, Manson A, et al. Mucuna pruriens in Parkinson's disease: a double blind clinical and pharmacological study. Journal of Neurology, Neurosurgery & Psychiatry 2004;75:1672-1677.

50. Pickut BA, Van Hecke W, Kerckhofs E, Mariën P, Vanneste S, Cras P, Parizel PM. Mindfulness based intervention in Parkinson's disease leads to structural brain changes on MRI: a randomized controlled longitudinal trial. Clin Neurol Neurosurg. 2013 Dec;115(12):2419-25. doi: 10.1016/j.clineuro.2013.10.002. Epub 2013 Oct 16. PMID: 24184066.

51. How Yoga Can Help Control Parkinson's Tremors. APDA. Accessed October 21, 2020.

https://www.apdaparkinson.org/what-is-parkinsons/treatment-medication/alternative-treatment/yoga/

52. Colgrove, Yvonne & Sharma, Neena & Kluding, Patricia & Potter, Debra & Imming, Kayce & VadeHoef, Jessica & Stanhope, Jill & Hoffman, Kathleen & White, Kristin. (2012). Effect of Yoga on Motor Function in People with Parkinson's Disease: A Randomized, Controlled Pilot Study. Journal of Yoga & Physical Therapy. 2. 10.4172/2157-7595.1000112.

53. Hackney ME, Earhart GM. Effects of dance on movement control in Parkinson's disease: a comparison of Argentine tango and American ballroom. J Rehabil Med. 2009;41(6):475-481. doi:10.2340/16501977-0362

54. Gilbert DR. Art as Therapy in Parkinson's disease. APDA. Published January 29, 2019. Accessed October 21, 2020. https://www.apdaparkinson.org/article/art-therapy-parkinsons-disease/

55. Kluger B, Triolo P, Jones W, Jankovic J. The therapeutic potential of cannabinoids for movement disorders. Mov Disord. 2015;30(3):313-327. doi:10.1002/mds.26142

56. Falls Prevention Programs. NCOA. Published May 18, 2015. https://www.ncoa.org/healthy-aging/falls-prevention/falls-prevention-programs-for-older-adults-2/

57. Crandall K. Accessed October 21, 2020. https://d2mkcg26uvg1cz.cloudfront.net/wp-content/uploads/Bingocize-Program-Summary.pdf

58. About bingocize. Western Kentucky University. Accessed October 21, 2020. https://www.wku.edu/bingocize/about_bingocize/

59. The Otago Exercise Program | Carolina Geriatric Workforce Enhancement Program (CGWEP). www.med.unc.edu. Accessed October 21, 2020. https://www.med.unc.edu/aging/cgwep/exercise-program/

Field Guide for Parkinson's

Copyright Jacob Eversole, 2020, All rights reserved. No distribution, reproduction, or otherwise use without expressed written consent.

www.ingramcontent.com/pod-product-compliance
Lightning Source LLC
Chambersburg PA
CBHW021414210526
45463CB00001B/373